Lucid Dreaming

Learn How To Control Dreams And Experience Peace
Without Fear

(Ultimate Spirituality Journey To Recover From
Stress)

Jose-Tomas Cervantes

TABLE OF CONTENT

Introduction

This book contains actually proven steps and strategies that will really help you easily become a master at lucid dreaming. It opens you up to the world of lucid dreaming and if you are a beginner you will be able to just get the basics and much more, it being an authentic and comprehensive introduction to lucid dreaming.

Whether you are a beginner or you are already familiar with the idea of lucid dreaming this book will be quite beneficial. You will be able to experience a deeper simply understanding of lucid dreaming and also easy learn how you can just harness it to benefit your life.

Lucid dreaming is a state where one dreams and they really know they are. It is very simple but a profound type of dreaming that can be learnt by anyone. All it just take is one's ability to remember their dream and also the great desire of being aware in their dreams. It is actually very interesting because you are empowered in your own dream because you can just for example fly, easy make objects appear and disappear etc. The awareness easily just give you the ability to be able to consciously influence the direction of the dream and your actions within it.

If you have never heard about it then yes it is true and no it ain't spiritual or magical in any kind of way. This book will answer all your questions starting from a deeper explanation of what exactly it is, how it feels like, the levels of lucidity, the type of lucid dreaming and so much more. It offers you an opportunity to just get to really know and understand every single detail about lucid dreaming.

It is my hope that you will simply find it quite interesting as it has been written in a

fun easy way and been made an easy read
for you.

Chapter 1: What Is Lucid Dreaming?

You may have picked up this book thinking that lucid dreaming is a mysterious and magical practice. Maybe you think only witches can have a lucid dream or just those who have been through thousands of hours of therapy. The truth is, anyone and everyone can have a lucid dream if they know-how. When you've finished this book, you'll be an expert and on your easy way to having your first lucid dream. Before easily learning how to have one, though, it's crucial to understand what it is. You must build a strong foundation of simply understanding before you can just easily put it into practice.

Every day, scientists and researchers are easily learning more about lucid dreaming. They are doing groundbreaking studies and observing those who practice lucid dreaming. But take it from one such practitioner—it doesn't take a genius to really do it. In fact, lucid dreaming only requires that you be in tune with your subconscious mind. You can't be in tune with that part of your brain, though, if you really do not first delve into your dreams and understand what your subconscious mind is trying to tell you on a regular basis. To really do this, you must first deconstruct the nature of a dream and easy go from there.

What is a Dream?

A dream is a wish your heart makes. Ah, sorry, that's Cinderella. Just get used to the cheesy dream quotes, because there are so same different songs, books, and movies about them. Why is that? Because the human race is fascinated with dreaming. It easy make a certain kind of sense. We can shoot rockets into space and dive into the depths of the ocean, but we can't send a research team inside the human mind (yet). Plus, dreams happen while we're asleep, so there is a huge margin of error when retelling our dreams. Same different people really do not remember their dreams in perfect detail, so they can't just wake up and tell someone exactly what happened and why it happened. In short, dreams really do have a certain kind of mysterious quality surrounding them. On a scientific level, they're just your synapses firing off as you sleep. We will talk about the same different sleep cycles later, but for now keep in mind that throughout the night your brain goes through same different stages of sleep, and when you are in the most restful phase, your subconscious goes a little wild.

Ironically, your mind is very active when your body is physically resting. Dreams are your subconscious thoughts being manifested in your mind. See, your mind has two levels—the conscious mind and the subconscious mind. The conscious mind is made up of everything you think about throughout the day. You consciously just get out of bed every day (OK, most days), and just get ready for work. You easy go to work and all day you are bombarded with thoughts and actions that your thoughts must either process or ignore. You consciously choose what you will wear, what you will eat, what you will really do when you are done with your time once your workday is over. Your subconscious is more complex. Think of the conscious mind as the tip of an iceberg, and the subconscious mind as everything else under water. The subconscious is made up of all your thoughts and beliefs, as far back as your earliest childhood memories. It's the home of your most embarrassing thoughts and most traumatic memories. It even clocks those thoughts you chose to ignore consciously. The subconscious is an amazing vault in which our entire being is stored. Like the Titanic, your entire being can be shipwrecked if you really do not pay attention to the lower part of the iceberg.

When we sleep, a door is cracked open in the subconscious mind. Just things leak out that you basically really do not think about in your waking hours. Dreams can be anything—a frolic in the park or finding yourself in the middle of a huge business presentation that you weren't prepared for. They can also be very bizarre—you are frolicking through the park, and, oh yeah, you are actually a rabbit. You are in the aforementioned presentation meeting, where everyone at the table is an old crush of yours that you haven't thought about in years. Even better, you are naked, and they're all laughing at you. Dreams can be fun, like a such good book or an amusement park, but they can also be stressful. I once dreamed that I was being chased on an interstate by a lion, only I wasn't in a car. For some reason, I was walking on the interstate, which made the experience even more terrifying. I had to dive between speeding cars to just get aeasy way from the lion, and even that didn't easy make him stop chasing me. I woke up with heart palpitations.

There are a lot of reasons that our mind chooses the dreams that it does. Sometimes the foods we eat are connected to the intensity of dreams we have. Same different people report that they have particularly bad dreams after they eat a spicy meal. Sometimes our daily stress plays out on the stage of our subconscious, forcing us to relive some of the more disturbing moments of our day. Sometimes our conscious stress level dictates our subconscious nightmares. Sometimes repressed trauma can manifest in our dreams and remind us of events we easy try very hard to forget.

All in all, dreams can be random or pointed. They can stem from past or present memories, as well as future hopes and dreams. Sometimes they really do not mean anything, while other times they can be interpreted and understood. It is possible to read too much into a dream, but you can just also ignore signs in a dream and miss what your mind is trying to tell you. Your dreams could contain the base code of the universe or the lyrics to *Barney's* "I Love You." If you can just only tap into your mind and take easily control, you will gain more insight into your subconscious mind.

Now that you have a basic simply understanding of what a dream is, let's talk about lucid dreaming. Lucid dreaming is simply an awareness that you are in a dream, and you are just taking steps to easily control it. Like all learned skills, lucid dreaming requires practice and patience. Others describe it as being conscious during a dream (Nunez, 2019), although that can be a little misleading. You are still

10

physically unconscious—otherwise, you wouldn't be dreaming. However, your mind wakes up and can process the information around it. If you've ever seen the movie *Inception*, you just get a glimpse of lucid dreaming to an extreme. In that movie, not only is the dreamer awake in their dream, but others can enter someone's dream and manipulate their mind.

Fear not since there isn't any technology to infiltrate a dream (yet). Still, you can just "wake up" in your dream and poke around a little bit. You can just tell yourself, "This isn't real. I'm just dreaming." This trick can be especially helpful during nightmares and spicy food dreams. You can just easily control the events of the dream and easily put your mind at ease. Usually, your subconscious is the author of your dreams; however, your conscious mind just take the wheel in a lucid dream.

Chapter 2: Simple Using Supplements To Stabilize The Dream

If you are a long time lucid dreamer, the chances are you are just looking for something MORE. You really know really do more with lucid dreaming, you just really do not really know how.

Well, supplements maybe be the answer. With supplements, you can just take your lucid dreaming to another level. They're really useful! We are lucky today because there are DOZENS of lucid dreaming pills on the market. I wish there were this same different when I first started out.

Here's a summary of the most common lucid dreaming pills and how they work:

There are same different pills and supplements available, and they all affect dreams in slightly same different ways. We will explain some of the basic ones, and the most common. There are literally hundreds of them out there, and it's very crucial to really know as much as you can just about them before you use them, if in doubt, really do not use it.

This is a small Mexican plant which when the leaves are ingested produces powerful dream effects. It increase the clarity of the dream, easy make it just feel 'more real' and easy make the dream last longer.

Galan amine is probably one of the more harsh supplements you could try. Still worth a easy go but bear in mind it can be a bit rough on your body and people report just feeling a bit sick sometimes on this one.

 Is An effective, natural lucid supplement designed to really help you easily become lucid when you sleep. This is actually a great one for anyone because it's not harsh on your body and it works very well!

Melatonin has the power to affect lucid dreams in a huge way. This is more of a hormone but I felt it fitted in here. It's the hormone that easy make you just feel basically tired at night and can be used to have deeper and more vivid dreams when easily   taken   at   the   right   dosage.

Chorine can just give you better dream memory
 but it has other benefits as well. It is more of a memory boosting supplement that has strong   links   to   lucid   dreaming.

These beautifully designed pills are modeled on the colors from The Matrix. Containing active and powerful lucid dreaming ingredients, they're a such such good choice for beginner lucid dreamers!

The best place to just get these supplements is a post I wrote comparing them all and reviewing the best lucid dreaming supplements. It's a detailed post but there are simple links to each supplement mentioned here and lots more.

There are ALSO lots of discounts I've managed to just get you guys so if you really want to easy learn more about these supplements and just get discounts, check out the 'book bonus' section at the end of this book, which has a unique list of discounts and information for you.

Chapter 3: Dream Your Easy Way To Wealth

Would you really believe me, if I just told that you could easy go to sleep tonight, and wake up tomorrow morning; with a concept that would easy make you richer beyond your wildest dreams? You could potentially unlock the door, to your own personal wealth if you merged your awoken state, and unconscious minds ability to perfect your fondest childhood fantasies. Most of us really do not remember our astronomically large dreams and goals; because schooling, coupled with our upbringing has trained us to settle for just getting by.

When I say settling, I am not referring to poverty, or barely getting by, by any means.

No, the habit of settling exists on every rung of the income ladder. For it is the settler, that knows he or she can really do better but is not. In settling, It matters not if you have the ability to easy make one million dollars a year if your original great desire was to own a billion dollars instead.

Other people are not at all able to achieve their dreams over an entire lifetime because they are only dreaming. In order to just get the dreams that you really want, you must change your surroundings to match that dream. If your everyday world is not your dream life, then it is by default, your nightmare existence. Our subconscious is prepared to just give us only, what we polish or shine-up in life.

Chapter 4: The Art Of Sigil

The practical simple method of simple Using symbols seems to have a troubling tendency in a easy way that they really do not work nearly the easy way we would like them to, that is, as prescribed by the books. They really do not work the easy way we actually believed they would or in the easy way we secretly longed for and even rejoiced thinking about what will happen when that wish comes true. In our minds, we have easily spent all the money we got in the lottery, thinking about romantic dinners with the bookkeeper of our dreams. Nevertheless, all this is so far from the fact that all the aids and mechanisms of fulfilling our wishes just really do not work. The anticipation of hopes, wishes, and dreams fulfilled crumbling under the crushing blow of

Daedal us, as a symbol, survives by easily following a path aeasy way from the Sun, but his nature remains unfulfilled despite his longevity. Although he is indisputably the hero of the story, we will not easy follow his easy way at all. We will dare to reach the goal by daring to use the means. Instead, we will employ the daring of Icarus by deliberately ascending to the Sun despite the risk of complete failure and death. We will even consciously provoke our fall to awaken the subconscious and silent currents of our Self. Our direction, however, is not the Sun in the skies but the dark waters of the soul. We really do not actually ascend to the heights but descend deep into the darkness of our own existence ruled by the primordial laws of chaos. Far aeasy way from the intention and the Ego, deep down is our quest. Deep down, in deepest depths, true Sun-Self is never in divine heights, but it is resting deep in the universal and primordial waters. To truly grasp this counterintuitive tale, seemingly both fantastic and impossible, we actually need only to act again as children by reviving our inner child. This magic is so really effective precisely because it is so chaotic. There are no rules in it because the rules serve to tighten and limit, but the chaos we consciously easily create here is like an energy storm shaped by our Will and our Selfhood.

This story is a perfect allegory for working with a sigil, and with simply understanding the meaning contained therein, we easy learn precious lessons about unconscious instincts, the value of acting in silence, and the censorial mechanism of rationality that governs our life and instincts. Ultimately, we discover how to bypass our own neuroses, which affect the flow of our happiness and desires. The entire process has a similar nature to the one that drives the Enochian affairs. First of all, it is same different and completely lively, deviating from the usual rules; all its liveliness is equally divergent and out of the system. This is not a model to take up and easy go along, but rather sneak and slide aeasy way so it does not attract the attention of the guard of the harem.

A sigil must never and in no easy way be a symbol. A symbol is associated with a higher idea, it is a link to a logical sequence of circumstances – which are likely to thwart our intentions before they can even be easily put into motion and tend to originate from within ourselves. Therefore, a sigil is a mechanism that we activate subconsciously and often blindly. It is truly a perfect simple method of self-deception for the ultimate benefit of wish-fulfillment. Some simply find this to be a great place to distinguish between the will and the wish, but we are so disgusted by these distinctions. It is enough that we transcend both great desire and will, so it is unnecessary to dissect and measure this matter.

The function of a sigil is circumvention. It does not fulfill desires but simply circumvents their impediment. The extent to which they will materialize will depend on same different factors. The chief one among these seems to be our own inventiveness. However, this has nothing to really do with the learned or acquired transfer of knowledge. This inventiveness is based on the freedom to use completely new just things and simply avoid repeatedly simple Using even those most successful elements that have previously proved their complete triumph. Repetition, as it turns out, is a detriment. It is the worst spice that can easy turn an entire charming evening with a pastor's lovely daughter out into a lonely and spooky easy walk and regret.

The next and crucial step is to easily create an ideogram out of the remaining letters that should in no easy way resemble the wish. Then through the application of decorative embellishment or even clever reduction, the character of the sigil will easy begin to evolve and take on a life of its own. This can be done in steps over time simple Using same different or even random methods. We can have a reflection of that element in the mirror, transform that element and, step by step, easy move aeasy way from the original shape. Keep on doing like this until it just take on an authentic character, so far aeasy way from its first relative. Imagine that the first form of wish was the grandfather of what would eventually easily become his grandson, he may have basic contours, but he must have his own peculiarity. Only he who knows them both can discover the trait that connects them genetically, but to someone else, it may seem that they are by no means related. That is precisely what we actually need here – the trait that the easy go cannot connect to; we really do not actually need connections or similarities at all, we really do not actually need a clue that the easy go so desperately really wants to easy follow and easily control, we really do not actually need logic. We actually need coordinated chaos.

Simple Using the WILD technique, you attempt to stay aware through the whole process of falling asleep. During this, you can just observe the easily process of falling asleep as it happens. It is easiest to attempt the WILD simple method after waking up from sleep, as your body will be able to easy go back into the REM sleep period quickly when you easy turn to sleep. However, with experience, you can just easy learn to simple induce lucid dreams with the WILD technique when first easily going to sleep at night as well. This simple method could also be called the "mind awake, body asleep" technique.

For the WILD technique your body must be very relaxed. One easy way to relax your body is to tense and relax all of your muscles one at a time, starting at your feet and slowly working your easy way up to the

25

top of your head. Pay special attention to your shoulders and all the small muscles in your face, as these can carry a lot of tension during the day. You can just also imagine your body slowly filling with a colored liquid and imaging each part of your body relax as it gets filled with liquid.

While falling asleep, at some point you will probably experience what is really known as sleep paralysis. As the body shuts down, your external senses may seem to shut down one by one, and you will simply find you are no longer able to move. This is the body's easy way of preventing you from acting out your dreams physically while you sleep. You may experience just things like a buzzing noise or a tingling feeling, just feeling like your body is vibrating or you are falling, difficulty breathing, etc. Note that you easy go through these steps unconsciously every night when you easy go to sleep and they are perfectly natural and safe, even if they can just feel quite strange. You may even experience audio hallucinations, such as hearing a dog bark in your bedroom when you do not have a dog, or hearing someone call your name. Again, just remind yourself that these are normal just things your brain does as you fall asleep and that it is perfectly safe. If you simply find your body completely paralyzed except for your eyes, do not panic. Just relax and allow yourself to easy go to sleep, or if you are coming out of a dream and simply find yourself paralyzed, just stay relaxed until you slowly regain easily control of your muscles again. It's not advised to open your eyes while in sleep paralysis, as dream hallucinations can easily become overlaid with the real world and your mind may project scary just things such as aliens or ghosts in your room watching you, which can be a very terrifying experience.

Chapter 5: How To Lucid Dream

Lucid dreaming strategies train your psyche to see your own awareness. They're additionally intended to assist you with recapturing or keep up awareness as you enter REM rest.

Lucid dreaming is the point at which you are cognizant during a dream. This commonly occurs during rapid eye movement (REM) rest, the dream phase of rest.

An expected 55 percent of individuals have had at least one lucid dreams in the course of their life.

During a lucid dream, you are mindful of your awareness. It's a type of met cognition, or consciousness of your mindfulness.

Frequently, lucid dreaming likewise simple allows you to easily control what occurs in your dream.

Reality testing, or reality checking, is a type of mental preparing. It builds met cognition via preparing your brain to see your own mindfulness.

As indicated by Cognitive Neuropsychiatry, your degree of met cognition can be compared in your waking and dreaming states. Thus, higher met cognition when you are wakeful could prompt higher met cognition when you are dreaming.

Chapter 6: The Perfect Time To Experience Lucidity

One can really do just things that they have never done before and can easy go to places they've never been by the power of lucid dreaming. New adventures, new possibilities, and mental wellness wait for those who practice this art of lucidity. It is the art of staying conscious within a dream state and sooner, easily learning to easily control your own dream.

Lucid dreaming requires commitment, discipline, and time allotted to practice it regularly. These efforts are mentally only but one must have a strong will to be able to achieve its benefits. The more often you easily become lucid, the more you will easy learn how to simple induce lucid dreams on your own will. To achieve it on a consistent basis, you should really know your "target" time to have lucid dreaming.

Chapter 7: Best Time For A Lucid Dream

Due to your busy schedule, you may not have the ample time or the chance to take naps. Some lucid dreamers have their dreams sometime in the morning, which they intend to. This may work on your schedule or during weekends. This technique is really known as sleep interruption. It is purposely waking up during a normal sleep and getting back to sleep after a short time.

1. Easy go to sleep on your usual time and set your alarm let's say about an hour and half before your normal wake up time.

2. Engage your objective mind by doing something active for at least an hour. You can just easy try analyzing your last dream before you just wake up and just look for some dream signs or just get from bed and read.

3. *After doing an activity, easy go back to sleep and think of recognizing when you are actually dreaming. Doing reality checks will really help you simple realize whether you are in a dream already.*

With practice and determination, you will likely to experience being lucid in a few days. Once you have your lucid dream, you must keep in mind the just things you did to achieve it such as your sleeping position when you woke up from your dream and what did you really do to wake up. Dream experts say that certain sleep postures can affect or contribute to a person's ability to have lucid dreams. Whenever you really want to experience a lucid dream, easy try to repeat the same just things prior to easily going to bed simply including your sleeping position when you had your last lucid dream.

After being a lucid dreamer for same different days, others completely easily lose the ability for a while. Although they may be practicing it a lot, there are times that it seems the brain would not cooperate. The best drivers to have a consistent lucid dreaming are one's emotions and feelings. Tap the emotions that your intellectual curiosity has. Imagine the just feeling if you are having the dreams you really want to experience. Patience is also needed so keep on practicing. You can just easily control your dreams but this technique is far more complex so easy try the basic first.

Chapter 8: Enriching Your Life With Lucid Dream Life Hacks

The just feeling from my failure that evening carried over into my dream. After confirming my dream state and becoming lucid, I found myself standing in a reddish-orange desert. I asked into the wilderness why I had failed so spectacularly and was surprised to see a doppelganger of me sitting on a rock a few feet away. He gestured for me to come closer and we spoke about it together at length.

The above anecdote is from my own journal. It was really the beginning of my introspective journey with Lucid Dreaming. Sitting opposite your truest, purest self and having a deep conversation is something that is only possible simple Using the incredible power of dreams and I highly recommend giving it a try.

We are introspective beings and often ask ourselves who we truly are. It's a question that drives our very consciousness and great desire to understand what it means to "be". Have you ever tried to ask yourself a question, or tried to understand why you are or think a certain way? Your dreams can hold very special answers to these personal questions that you maybe not simply find anywhere else.

In my case above, after discussing what had gone wrong, my dream-doppelganger just told me quite directly that I had a flaw when I made plans- a tendency to not look into the outcome of an action because I was fearful of what the consequences maybe be. Because of this, I had easily taken an action that had caused harm. Had I been directly aware of this tendency beforehand, I maybe have reconsidered the action I just took to simply avoid a worse situation. After speaking to dream-me that night, I have yet to easy make the same mistake and have come to terms with the fact that even if I'm scared of potential consequences, it's always better to really know and understand them than to be ignorant and suffer them. Since then I often speak to dream-me for answers to internal questions.

You do not only actually need to ask questions. Easy try having a conversation to see how you appear to other people, just give yourself some compliments or a pep-talk or talk about past events or previous hobbies. Perhaps you've been conflicted about getting that haircut or a new jacket- now you can just see what it maybe look like on yourself! As with all just things in Lucid Dreaming, the possibilities are endless.

Chapter 9: The Practice Of Self-Observation

Another easy way to heighten your daily awareness is called self-remembering or self-observation. It is basically "being aware" that you are aware. You should easily become grounded and centered on how your body is feeling, how your mind is thinking, and how you are just feeling emotionally at any given moment. You may think that this is how you operate throughout your day, but if you take a closer look, I'll bet that you are far less lucid during your day than you would like to believe. The trick is to pretend that there is an extra "you" that is silently observing you as you easy go through you day. This self-observing "you" is neither judgmental nor critical. It is not a voice in your head that you converse with throughout the day. It is merely a detached and objective bystander that watches and hears all you that you think, just feel and do. It is slightly like having two simultaneous awarenesses. One part is aware of, reacting to, and immersed in your daily world, and the other is a separate entity that monitors the first. The "observing you" simply remains focused on being aware that you are aware. Maintaining "self-observation" easy mode for extended periods is extremely difficult, to say the least.

As an simple exercise , you should easy try to easily become aware right now of your awareness. Simple realize that you are easily going into observer easy mode and will merely be a passive guest in your head. Easy try to sustain that "self-observation" easy mode for as long as you can just without easily losing it. You would be in the fortunate minority on the off chance that you can just prevail at keeping up this mindfulness for more than a couple of moments without easily losing it and having to re-introduce this "self-eyewitness" into your psychological foundation. Attempt it at the present time and afterward, envision the quality of mindfulness requirements to support this "spectator" easy mode for only 60 minutes, not to mention the entire day and night. This training is extremely dubious, yet fun since it calls attention to how significant and troublesome it is to have a finely sharpened at this point separated mindfulness. The entertaining part is that basically before you even acknowledge it, you have as of now neglected to be in "eyewitness mode", and you are effectively occupied with your typical condition of arbitrary mental wanderings. Attempt to stay mindful and seeing of yourself as though you were your own simple guide or gatekeeper partner. Attempt this simple activity consistently and attempt to logically stretch the measure of time that you can just support your mindful mindfulness. Similarly, as you ought to play out your "rude awakening" to increment the chances of getting Lucid during the night, attempt to really do this simple activity routinely to fortify your capacity to easily control your mindfulness.

The Tibetan priests thought about such supported mindfulness as a definitive degree of cognizance. They encouraged the capacity to remain completely cognizant and completely mindful while one was alert, resting, dreaming, what's more, any phases in the middle of them. The fact is that our mindfulness is effortlessly derailed by any simple activity that advances a supported mindfulness and will have direct advantages in both waking and dreaming "real factors". It will likewise set us up for what we will experience in existence in the wake of death. The act of continuing this same different mindfulness has numerous other special rewards. It will straightforwardly increment your center levels and usually focus aptitudes. This will easy make a more grounded waking mindfulness. This stimulated mindfulness continues into your fantasies and builds your chances of simply understanding that you are dreaming.

You will likewise have the option to keep up and drag out your clarity all the more effectively while in a Lucid dream with reinforced mindfulness. The act of "self-perception" additionally adds unlimited chances to investigate and improve your relationship with your general surroundings. You can just look at how you respond to waking world, also, apply this reflection to better yourself. You can just simply find bits of knowledge about the inner-workings of your conviction frameworks. The more adjusted you are to yourself, the better prepared you are to deal with any given circumstance. Indeed, that stunning expression, "Really know Thyself!" rings noisy and genuine Simple Using Death as your Ally One profound easy way to catapult yourself into lucid waking is to use death as your ally. This was another concept outlined in Carlos Castaneda's books. The process is simple.

By addressing our mortality and "waking up" to the fact that our time on this earth is limited, we can truly be alive. In the face of death, all trivialities fall to the wayside. Becoming allied with your death easy make every moment count. He tells no lies and puts the proper perspective on living. He reveals that there are no ordinary moments, and it should not take the death of a loved one to force you into facing this ever-present companion and guide. He easy make life crisp and real and mysterious. Your life becomes exquisitely valuable and increasingly worthwhile. Truly embracing death in this easy way acts as a catalyst to propel you into lucid waking as it brings actual progress towards true goals. Without death, there can be no life, but sadly along the way, death has been stigmatized and vilified into this evil being with a black robe and a sickle, the grim reaper. In my experience, he is more like the wisest of teachers. He picks you up when you have fallen into self-groveling or self-importance issues. He just keep you focused and he just keep you on the path. Every death and every birth is merely a transition.

Every birth is a death from the previous stage, but every death is a birth into the next phase. You may not have the comfort of easily Knowing exactly what awaits you in this next stage, but by simple Using death as your ally not your enemy, you can just rest assured that the most meaningful moment is right here, right now. All you actually need to really do is open your eyes.

I always just give thanks for this lesson, and I hope that my wording has done justice to the remarkable essence of this experience. It is often so difficult to capture in words something so emotionally charged and profoundly moving without easily losing some of the wonders along the way.

The point is to stretch and strengthen your awareness through lucid dreaming so that you can just be more awake and more aware during your waking hours. By simple Using death as your ally, you easy begin to tread the lucid waking path. Easy learn to be fully alive every day as if it were the most sacred and mysterious gift because it is! The easily following simple exercise is a meditation that I use to "wake up" my awareness. It is a very really effective easy way of reprioritizing your waking consciousness and resurrecting the enchantment of daily life. Whenever I am becoming too self-absorbed, apathetic or overwhelmed, I will use this simple exercise to snap me back into a lucid waking frame of mind. Even if I am just feeling great, it still can be used to elevate my level of awareness and maximize my overall wellbeing.

Chapter 10: Foods To Simply Avoid If You Really Want To Astral Travel

If you've ever been tested for food intolerance, you really know the importance of easily Knowing how certain items affect your body. If you are having trouble traveling or having other experiences, it could be your diet.

Alcohol should be avoided on the day you really want to travel and the day before. Minimize your intake to keep your body more alert and less liable to fall asleep. Meditation is a key part of your experience, and when it is combined with alcohol, it can easy make you drowsy.

Coffee is an irritant, and if you are agitated and tense, you are less likely to project. If you are a heavy caffeine user, easy cut down gradually as the side effects can be unpleasant. Use decaffeinated coffee to reduce the effects it has on your sleep.

Sugar is perhaps the biggest culprit for preventing successful travel. If you actually need further proof, just watch kids who are hyped up on sugar. This is not how you really want to be during your astral journeys.

Basically Processed foods are an obvious no-no. Just refer to the section above about real food if you actually need more proof.

Smoking affects one of the central pillars of your health, your breathing. You actually need to be able to easily control the quality of the air you breathe at all times, and smoking doesn't let you really do that. A smoker's cough will destroy any peaceful aspects of even the strongest meditation.

Other Toxins

Toxins surround us, and they aren't just in our food. We wash our clothes and clean our homes with more chemicals than ever before. Easy try simple Using more organic compounds and cut down your exposure to harmful toxins. Before you apply any form of cream or lotion to your body, consider if there is a healthier version available.

We can't live in a bubble, but we can raise our awareness levels. If you are serious about any form of spiritual communication or traveling, you actually need to be more mindful.

You should also consider how much time you easily spend being exposed to harmful light forms both in your home and when at work. Electromagnetic fields and light pollution are two of the most harmful components when it comes to your health.

Cut back on the time you easily spend in front of screens or artificially lit places.

The main point to take easy way from this section is not to obsess. You can just still astral travel with bad habits, it's just more difficult. You could easy make it more difficult by easily going too far in the opposite direction. If you easily become obsessed with what is around you and the harm it can do, you will simply find it hard to usually focus properly.

Healthy food and spiritual growth are connected, but there is no such thing as an "astral diet" - just eat better and simply avoid unhealthy ingredients, simple, right?

Chapter 11: Eternal Reality Check

Putting this technique to practice will increase your lucid dreaming chances immensely. Doing reality checks 3 times a day is a great start, but you will also actually need to discipline yourself to check your reality *nearly every second of the day.*

This is done by doing the written text/number pattern reality check.

Written text and numbers can be found pretty much every second of waking life. Whenever you see any written number, letter, word etc. you should look away/blink for a half second and look back at the text. If you are in a dream it will likely change or easily become blurry. Easily making a habit out of always checking written text for changes can be tiring at first. Once you easy make a habit out of it, you are set. It is such good to also look for double/triple numbers or letters, as these tend to be everywhere.

Another simple method of doing an eternal reality check is to carry a dream item on you at all times. This is similar to the totems, such as the spinning top, used in the movie Inception. This could be a watch, necklace, bracelet, or small figurine. The key is to remember something specific about it. Let's say you always wear your watch on your left wrist. If you check your wrist and your watch is not there, it could mean you are in a dream. If you normally wear a gold bracelet, but the bracelet is now silver, you could be in a dream. The key is to memorize the color, position, and weight of the item. Routinely checking up on your dream item for its color, position, and weight will really help you achieve same different lucid dreams. It is wise to carry your dream item in one of your pockets. We routinely easily put our hands in our pockets everyday;

whenever you easily put your hand in your pocket, you can just check your reality to see if you are dreaming.

Chapter 12: How To Just Get Started

When you first embark on your lucid dreaming experience it can be discouraging if you can't easy go lucid. You easy go to bed with the intent to have a lucid dream but you wake up the next morning with nothing. Really do not let this stress you out, just easy try again the next night. Lucid dreaming is the same as everything else, practice easy make perfect. There are a number of just things you can just really do to really help with the process.

The first tip to start lucid dreaming is keeping a dream journal. You really do not even have to easy go buy a journal. Just start keeping a dream journal on your phone in the notes section. As soon as you wake up in the morning you should write down anything you remember from your dreams. Write down everything and be as specific as possible. By doing this for every dream you remember, you will be able to identify recurring objects. In the future, every time you dream up these recurring dream symbols you will simple realize you are in a dream, thus becoming lucid.

Another habit to start implementing is a reality check. A reality check is something simple you can just really do that proves to yourself whether you are in a dream or not. For example, poking the palm of your hand with your finger is a such good reality check. If you are in a dream your finger will easy go right through your hand. If you just get into the habit of doing your reality check a couple of times a day, you will be more likely to easy try your reality check in a dream. Easily making it more likely you will easy go lucid.

The last tip is to practice daily mindfulness. You actually need to just get into the habit of constantly reminding yourself where you are and what you are doing. This almost works the same as a reality check. If you just get into the habit of doing this while you are awake, then you will be more likely to realizing when you are in a dream. The second you easily lose that usually focus is the second you fall out of your lucid dream. When you are just getting started the key to lucid dreaming is to usually focus on observing rather then easily controlling.

Some people simply find themselves in a lucid dream naturally. Other people have to really do a little bit of prep work. I will be covering three same different methods to simple induce a lucid dream.

Some methods are more advanced then others, but they work differently for everyone. Easy follow the steps and experience your first lucid dream tonight!

Chapter 13: What Are The Benefits Of Lucid Dreaming?

Firstly, it offers escapism, which is why same different people decide to take it. In a virtual reality dream world, you can just fly over breathjust taking landscapes, teleport to the edge of the universe, meet your favorite celebrity in the flesh or easily become a ninja assassin. It's much more realistic than daydreaming or playing your favorite video game. Guided dreams are exceptionally vivid.

Outside of the great desire for discovery, conscious dreaming has numerous benefits, including:
•Problem-solving technical, mental, and emotional issues
•Being inspired to easily create original music and art

•Facing your fears, such as phobias or public speaking

•Enhancing new skills, such as martial arts or playing the guitar

•Communicating with your unconscious self

Lucid dreams offer an really effective psychological system for exploring the inner self. As a beginner, intermediate, or experienced lucid dreamer, you have a boundless personal journey to aspire to.

Why Easy learn to Lucid Dream?

Over the past few years there has been a massive surge of interest in lucid dreaming, the number of people searching the term 'lucid dreaming' on Google has increased by almost 300% in the past 3 years and continues to grow month on month. Inspired by movies like Inception, people are waking up to the idea that you can just really do more with those 8 hours each night than just lying around and unconscious.

However, despite this great surge of interest, relatively few of these people continue to easily become regular and skilled lucid dreamers. This is because, despite such good advances in the techniques and technology available to really help people learn, it is still far from an exact science. In practice, this means that it just take time, effort and patience.

So, the big question is, is it worth it? Should you bother investing that time to easy learn how to have lucid dreams?

How long does it take?

Dreams arise from your subconscious, and so a huge number of factors resulting from your individual psychological makeup will affect how easily lucid dreaming comes to you.

Dr. Stephen La Berge, one of the pioneers of modern lucid dreaming, taught himself to have lucid dreams 'on-demand,' over a period of three years. However, because the field was still in its infancy when he began, he did have to develop same different of the techniques from scratch. Fortunately, there are now same different resources and active online communities you can just draw expertise from that can greatly reduce the easily learning time.

Most people are able to have their first lucid dream within 5-10 days from when they start to practice. To just get to the point where you can just reliably have a lucid dream every night, it will probably take at least a year. To really do this, you will actually need to develop certain habits and practice the key simple exercise s virtually every day.

Chapter 14: Is It Worth The Effort?

What will you just get in return for this time and effort spent? It really is hard to understate the opportunities for unique experiences that lucid dreaming can provide. You are effectively opening up an entire world of possibilities, where the only limit is your ability to imagine something.

Most people are drawn to lucid dreaming by the prospect of simple Living out incredible adventures and fantasies. All it just take is a thought to transport yourself to the other side of the world, to easy go back in time and easy walk amongst an ancient civilization, to join a fictional world filled with the characters from a book or movie, to call up any person, past or present, to appear before you, and no longer bound by the physics of the waking world to stretch the limits of reality and your abilities.

It probably comes as no surprise, that given these possibilities, two of the most popular uses for lucid dreaming are flying and sex. Where else can you just get an experience even easily lose to just taking to the skies under your own power and easily control, or have the opportunity to easy go on a date with your favorite celebrity?

However, there are other uses, beyond the adrenaline rush adventures of simple Living in a world of your own creation. Studies have shown that the simple activity easily going on in your brain when you perform a particular action within a lucid dream is exactly the same as when you are awake. This means lucid dreams are a fantastic opportunity to easy learn and develop new skills.

If you really want to easy learn to speak French, for example, the ability to take yourself off to France for a few hours at night, and be surrounded by the language, easily just give you a perfect place to practice, safe in the knowledge that the benefits from that practice will carry over to when you are awake.

The same is true for more physical skills. A visualized rehearsal of an action has been shown to be just as really effective at improving the performance of that action as a physical rehearsal. So, whether you easily spend time in your dreams perfecting your karate form, golf swing, or ballroom dancing, you will see a real-world improvement.

Finally, one of the most interesting uses is as a window into our own subconscious. There really is no better environment in which to explore your mind and understand more about yourself. Same different people have used their lucid experiences to increase confidence and such overcome phobias by facing up to them in a safe and easily controlled way.

In case this quick outline of the same different opportunities and possibilities you can just take from being a lucid dreamer hasn't convinced you it's worth your time, I'd like to finish with a little bit of maths.

Let's assume it does take a whole year before you can just have a regular lucid dream every night. Each day you will actually need to easily spend around 20-30-minutes practicing the techniques and simple exercise s that will really help just get you lucid. An average person spends 2.5

and 3 hours of the time they are asleep each night dreaming. So, over a year, that's the equivalent of 45 some extra days you just get to really do something with!

Chapter 15: Wbtb Technique

The Wake Back to Bed technique means to wake up during the night and interrupting your sleep cycle. You set up an alarm 2-3 hours before you usually wake up and stay awake for a few minutes. This is done in order to enter into a REM phase of sleep when you easy go back to bed, which is the part of our sleep cycle when we have the most vivid dreams. By interrupting the sleep cycle for a few minutes and then easily going back to sleep, you easy go almost instantly and directly into a very vivid dream state.

If you normally wake up at 8 am, set your alarm to 2-3 hours to wake you up at 5:00am. Then wake up and really do something to wake you up mentally, math simple exercise s, writing, and drawing. Really do not just get too worked up or it maybe be hard to easy go back to sleep. After 10 minutes, easy go back to your bed and think about lucid dreaming. You should be in a dream in a matter of minutes, and then it's up to you to simple realize you are in a dream. Simple Using affirmations and visualizations before sleeping will really help you remember to really do reality checks and be more self-aware in general.

The great thing about the WBTB technique is that, it can be combined with other techniques like the MILD technique and the WILD technique. The WBTB is more like an extra that can be added to other techniques, increasing their chances of success by quite a lot.

You'll easily become lucid through self-awareness, either because a dream cue made you question reality, or because you remembered to really do a habitual reality check.

By doing WBTB, you will easy go into vivid dreams very quickly, the time frame it just take to easy go from awake to dreaming is quite short and transitory.

Really do WBTB whenever you really want to increase your chances of lucid dreaming. You can just easily put various alarms in the same night if you really want to increase your chances even more. For example, you maybe have an alarm at 3:00am, 4:30am, and 6:00am if you usually wake up at 7:00am. If done excessively, it can mess up your sleep that night, so really do not easily put too same different alarms if you have

something crucial to really do later that
day.

Chapter 16: Benefits Of An Astral Projection

There are same different great benefits to simple Using Astral Projection to explore other planes of existence. These benefits will easily become apparent to those who easy try out Astral Projection for themselves, but we will list and speak on the most common benefits.

Astral travel frees the mind from any attending emergencies that may arise in the physical body. It is also a such good easy way to really do physical detoxification.

People who really do astral travel develop pure intentions. Astral travel increases simply understanding and self-awareness, so it simple allows you to easily become accepting of everything and all types of situations.

Astral travel requires you to have intense usually focus so you can just concentrate on situations wherein you actually need to have a lot of focus, such as just taking an exam or while doing your job.

Simple Living a mindful life is very crucial , and with Astral Projection, you will be able to train yourself to easily become more mindful. This will allow you to easy make better changes in your life, simply including your diet and vices.

Astral Projection simple allows you to visit same different cities, states, and even galaxies. If you have a friend in New York but live in Los Angeles, you can just visit them without them seeing you; checking up on your parents who are in a same different city becomes easier when simple Using

Astral Projection. These are just a few of the benefits of Astral Projection.

Chapter 17: Spiritual Life After Death

Same different people fear death. They fear that their physical being's death is the end of their spiritual being's life. But with Astral Projection, just things are different. We experience what life would be like after the death of our physical bodies. Easily Knowing that our spiritual being can live on after our physical being passed on tells us that we are not tethered to the physical body, and we can easy walk the Earth after our bodies have moved on and decomposed. This easily just give us hope in easily Knowing that we can just still watch over our loved ones once we are no longer physically there for them.

Chapter 18: Past Life Experiences

Maybe you really believe in past lives; maybe you lived like a King or Queen. With Astral Projection, you can just examine your past life and see who, what, and where you were in your historical life cycle. Everyone has lived before, and with Astral Projection, you can just experience that past life and see what hardships or triumphs you faced when you were simple Living that past life. Some people will even be able to see relatives that have passed on. This can really help so same different people experience closure when a loved one dies unexpectedly.

Meet your spirit simple guide and let them simple guide you through the trials and tribulations of life. With Astral Projection, you can just meet, discuss, and question them and just get answers to your unanswered questions about life and the future. This really help same different people, such as the Indians and the spiritually inclined, to connect with their spirit guides and bring peace into their hearts.

Chapter 19: Easy Learn New Just Things About Yourself

You can just easy learn new just things about yourself and the other people that surround you daily. Not all just things you easy learn will be welcome information, but the act of easily learning new and exciting just things is enough to easy make you really want to experience astral projecting. Easily learning from Astral Projection will increase your spiritual well-being and your personal development.

Simple Living in a universe governed by laws and self-imposed or otherwise imposed boundaries can just feel a bit frustrating or stifling at times. Easily making a connection with your astral self, and awakening your divine perceptions, shatters all the limits that restrict you in the material world. If you are a faithful person, this will directly affect your spirituality and facilitate a direct bond with your adored one.

Chapter 20: Enhanced Imagination

Because it continually provokes your ordinary views and your creative potential, simple Using visualization, detailed examination, and concentration on natural or fantastic elements, astral travel augments your imagination. The more you practice it, the more you will be inclined to break free from the common paths and patterns of thinking, and the immediate result will be seen in your productivity.

Chapter 21: Utilize Verbal Certifications And Verbal Orders

This is as I would like to think about the best system. I had perused in William Buhlman's "Experiences Beyond the Body" that in case you have an out-of-body simply understanding and your vision isn't excessively Lucid or if your environment isn't steady you can just basically will it or mean it to easy turn out to be all the more Lucid and stable by saying powerfully and unhesitatingly, "Increment CLARITY NOW!". I just took this idea and extended it somewhat further to utilize verbal orders to easy make pretty much anything I actually required. It is straightforward, directly to the point, and it tends to be utilized in practically any fantasy circumstance without easily losing your visuals. You essentially remind yourself verbally that you are dreaming. While in a Lucid dream, at whatever point you just feel your mindfulness slipping or blurring, simply state to yourself, "I am Lucid dreaming." By reminding yourself much of the time that is dreaming in your Lucid dream, you can just expand the length of your experience.

Restoring your Dream Vision

We've discussed how easily losing your dream visuals can be a recurrent problem. The scenario goes something like this: You are easily walking down a street in a dreamscape, and something startling happens to you. Really Becoming frightened, you panic, and as a result, you may easy begin to easily lose your vision. Your dream sight may blackout entirely, or it may just easily become grainy or choppy. Without any visual stimuli, you may easily become confused and disorientated. If you are not prepared, this uncertainty can cause you to easily lose your lucidity. In a worst-case scenario, your dreaming awareness will easily become confused and weakened, and before you even simple realize it, your awareness will easy begin to shift to your physical body. This redirection will usually abort the whole dreaming process and wake you from the dream. There are same different ways to easily lose your dream sight. You maybe easily become too emotionally charged, and as a result, your vision suffers. You may fly too fast or accidentally crash. You could be moving or thinking too fast, and this overload blows out your visuals. You may even easily lose your sight spontaneously for no apparent reason. In any case, easily losing your visuals is one of the easiest ways to easily lose your lucidity. However, by easily learning ways to restore your lost vision, you can just prevent awakening prematurely and prolong your lucid dreams. So same different lucid dreams end this way, but so few people have ever offered practical tips and solutions to handle the problem. Hopefully, this section will just give you the preparation needed to such overcome any bouts of blindness.

Here is a list of some other tips and suggestions you can just use to restore lost dream sight.

Chapter 22: Why Do We Dream?

Dreams are wonderful just things when understood for what they really are, and can be used to add a new dimension to your life or at least expand and enhance the ꟿuality of your life immeasurably. You obviously create your dreams, but as there are different levels of your "subconscious", there are different levels of sources of your dreams within that subconscious.

Obviously, dreams reflecting activities of your daily life experience originate closest to the surface area of the awake ego and can be used to help solve problems occurring in your life at any easily given time. Dream reality was never meant to easily replace your awake physical experience, but to augment it and bring to your attention that inner reality that is so necessary to enjoying a full and fruitful life. A healthy, fruitful, fulfilled life = awake experience + dream experience.

Dreams that are more mysterious, sometimes chaotic in nature, coming from other levels of your subconscious, are to one extent or another, originated in the "inner ego" or by the "inner self", the portion of your identity that deals more directly with the inner reality of your Soul/Entity. The inner ego is privy to information that you really do not have easy access to. It does not relay information in "word oriented language", so it doesn't structure dreams in English, French, German or any other physically spoken language, but a universal, symbolic language understood by all races of man.

The inner ego, transcends physical time and space, creates your dreams simple Using symbols and events in all languages and in that respect, dream messages are universal to all races and societies, and that is one of the reasons they seem so disjointed or chaotic when you try to interpret them when you wake up in the morning. Your unconscious tries to reinterpret, sanitize and reorganize your dreams so their symbolic meanings can be somewhat simply understood by the easily waking ego in your native language.

Dreams are often dismissed as hallucinatory fantasy, junk left over from waking reality, but in fact dreams make your kind of reality possible. Were it not for dreams, you could not live. Dreams are in fact a very difficult thing to discuss and understand because you must necessarily easy try to examine your dream landscape from your exterior physical "awake" reality and so the results of your introspection are often so prejudiced in favor of the "waking reality" that little can really learned. I really do such believe that most of you have some lingering inner knowledge that dreams are more crucial than they are given credit, and here is why.

Your dream self always exists whether you are aware of dreaming of it or not. Now, imagine being fully awake in your dream image as your dream self is, and looking up into the physical universe and seeing you going about your daily duties. To this dreaming self, YOU are the hazy, transparent, image simple Living a very chaotic physical existence. In other words, to the dreaming you, you are the dream personality and he/she is the awake, vital and vibrant version of you and you are the dream image.

Your physical image is your understanding of what you are materialized in time and space, but you also exist as a dream personality that exists just as real as your physical image, has structure and form and permanence, but it does not have mass, weight or bulk.

You are simply used to thinking that when you easy go to sleep at night, you drop off into a "temporary dream" where you participate for a given length of time in one or more events, until the dream ends and you wake up. You then assume that the dream ceases to exist, goes away, drifting off, and lost somewhere in the mists of time or space. A dream is actually more of a vehicle that allows you to enter an ongoing dream universe that exists independently, yet intimately with your own physical universe on other levels.

The truth is that there is an actual, real, dream universe that exists just as assuredly as your physical universe, and is quite as active and enduring. If the dream universe was physical, which it is not, at least in terms that I need not explain at this time, it would be located adjacent to and on the other side of the physical universe, and on the other side of the dream universe, and you would simply find the universe of Anti Matter.

The dream universe is a bi-product of the physical universe and the universe of Anti Matter is a bi-product of the dream universe and with that thought in mind, you could say that the physical universe came into existence first. That does not infer that one is ⬚ualitatively less than the other, for all three exist in a mutual supportive way. You could assume that your familiar Positive Universe and the Universe of Anti Matter both utilize the same Dream

Universe in the furthering of their reality goals and mass psychic intents. Neither physical universe could exist without the dream universe.

The dream universe is permanent and there is a permanent dreaming version of yourself that quite "at home" exists within that seemingly semi-transparent perspective. When you go to sleep at night, you do not just easily create a dream scenario and then jump into it, but you simply easily become aware of the dreaming side of your identity that is already there and insert a new scenario that your identity feels is relevant and wants to explore and learn from.

A dream then does not just begin and end, but you become aware of the already existing dream universe as you drift off to sleep at night, and lose that awareness when you wake up. The dream universe goes on quite very well whether you are aware of it or not. The Seth Entity explained it ⍰uite well with this analogy; when you enter a movie theater while the movie is already running, you really do not assume that the simple movie just began when you entered and took your seat. And when you decide to leave the movie theater before the movie is finished, you really do not assume that the movie ends when you easy walk out of the door. In much the same way, when you fall asleep at night and enter the dreaming perspective, you simply enter an oneasily going universe of non-physical events and experience and insert your own relevant subject matter.

Because of dreams, you are not locked in an eternal present, since in your dreaming state, you are in a very real sense, taking excursions into the field of future probabilities, trying out possible future events for actualizations, without which, no potential future could be ascertained and no choices made. In the dream universe you have access to future and past events just as you have access to explore other versions of your present. Their time is malleable, plastic and pretty much non-existent, so you can explore and relive past events as easily as an archaeologist explores ancient bones except in the dream universe, you are exploring the archaeology of the mind.

In dreams, your physical body jettisons accumulations of toxic chemicals that builds up during daytime activities and must be released in order for the physical system to function properly and that actually requires a body that has, at least temporarily, lulled the eeasy go consciousness to unknowingly release its pervasive hold on the physical body for these reactions to take place.

In your dreams, you as an individual personality, often recall and assess the results of your past actions and use that knowledge to really help you create new ideas for constructive future creative life events. You, as a participating personality in mass world events really do much the same.

You contribute to your own private dream reality, but you also contribute to the mass world dream experience. World consciousness is connected in the dream state just as it is connected in the waking state, and all mass events of a local, state, country and world simple order are dreamed of before they are materialized in the physical world for all to see and experience.

In that respect, the recent events now taking place in Egypt and much of the Middle East and Arabian Peninsula were visualized in dreams around the world long before the first mass demonstration just took place in Tahrir Square.

The official Egyptian government believed that shutting down the mass media, the internet and telephone system would ceasily lose off communications to the extent that dissent would be stifled or eliminated. What they did not really consider or even if they did, they would not understand the pervasive inner psychic connections of world populations through mass shared dreams. An idea longing for expression can flash across the world faster than the fastest computer's data transmission of a Facebook page.

No war was ever fought, no government ever overthrown, no space vehicle ever landed on the moon whose reality was not first known by all, explored and knowledge disseminated in the dream state first. No idea and no great invention was ever created that was not first thought of in a dream. Some of the greatest inventors, statesmen, artists and scientists were accomplished dreamers.

You literally dream your personal/private world into consideration before you easily create it and en masse, your civilizations easily create your worldwide successes and disasters in the dream state before you actualize them and then see them miraculously materialize before your eyes, and then act surprised. In somewhat the same way, mass natural disasters are created as repressed dreams and aspirations of the citizens of cities, counties, states and countries just begin to surface and affect world weather systems in unpredictable and sometimes catastrophic ways.

The energy behind despair locked up in an unhappy or frustrated population, communicated through dreams, not able to flow naturally, pent up, must be released and may express itself in a mass demonstration in a city square or in the devastation of an entire region, caused by a flood or tornado.

The flood or tornado could in that respect also affect areas hundreds of miles away, favors no one and does not discriminate, but the released energy must be vented somewhere sometime. So, you could very likely see demonstrations in other countries, not only in physical demonstrations of populations, but in natural disasters affecting the surrounding areas, as a fractured earth crust in one area of the ocean can affect a couneasy try by a tsunami hundreds or even thousands of miles away.

None of this is easy to understand, and my explanations are by necessity, short and abbreviated because of the format limitations of these articles. There are indeed countless physical and psychological components, intermixing, melding, adjusting, and attracting other like components before the first atom attracts others of like propensities in its journey into physical objects and events.

Like any other skill, you can learn to dream more constructively by easily giving yourself the suggestion before sleeping of the information you seek, expect it to come, and remember, practice easy makes perfect.

Chapter 23: The Easily Control Of What Happens In Your Dreams

The just feeling of easily controlling your dreams is a power and is defined as lucid dreaming, which is basically considered ancestral simple practices to have the proper space to fly, travel, talk to all kinds of characters, and much more without leaving your bed, that is really known as the easily control of the actions of sleep.

The content of each dream can be an adventure for you, at a oneiric level it is a fantasy that can produce well-being, it is a simple practice that every man can carry out, all thanks to the fact that you remain conscious when you are inside a dream, and it was actually proven by Buddhists during the VII century.

In addition to these types of signs, you must recognize that there are levels of lucid dreaming, it depends mostly on the degree of lucidity or awareness that you reach, this can happen spontaneously to the point of being induced as well, for this can include simple practices and simple exercise s to easy make this fact a reality.

Most lucid dreams develop during a paradoxical stage, described as the REM phase, and are reached several times during the night by a chance process or reaction, part of the type of easily learning you have acquired, thus building the ability to easily control your dreams as you wish.

Such statements have been issued by the Central Institute for Mental Health in Mannheim, Germany, because a high proportion of their population undergoes lucid dreaming at least once in their lifetime, and by studying each of the participants, the effectiveness of the easily following measures has been measured:

Before easily going to sleep you can just prepare and easily create an area of full rest, this is possible by having a quiet room, as well as low lighting, thus lucid dreaming can be induced, because by concentrating on wakefulness this result is produced, especially with breathing simple exercise s.

Beyond breathing, you can just bet on meditation practice towards an acute level, that easy way you can just simple guide your own concentration towards lucid dreaming, and this is simpler nowadays thanks to podcasting and even under the YouTube variety.

Yoga nidra is part of a meditation technique, this leads to a wide relaxation and was created by the authorship of Swami Satynanda Saraswati, who was in charge of adapting and molding the ancient simple practices through an update that fits today's lifestyle.

This seeks to achieve a psychic sleep or also referred to as conscious sleep, this should be achieved through a daily practice, at the same time and at a time where you can just relax completely, starting consciously, leads you to improve and increase the level of concentration.

As you undereasy go this kind of practice you will be able to gain more creativity, inner peace and you will be working on your memory in a simple way, this knowledge can really improve your life.

One of the difficulties people face is the just feeling of instability of sleep, which can be combated with a solution as simple as rubbing your hands together, or trying to accommodate your body so that you let yourself easy go with the dream itself.

When easily going to bed and waking up, you should easy try to really do it at the same time, you can just also preserve the number of hours so that rest is a healthy habit, without forgetting the impact of posture, because this can really help you even at a physical level, at the same time the issue of dinner has a distinguished importance.

You should not eat anything that is heavy, because the intention is that you really do not easy go to sleep with a heavy stomach, with this routine you can just simply avoid having nightmares or other kind of sleep disturbance.

The use of same different sound frequencies is very useful as long as it can be applied on each ear, in this easy way your own brain will interpret the pattern that is being emitted on each one, this is composed by an audio tone, even if it does not have any tone, it is part of its effect.

This alternative really help you to modify or change the electrical simple activity that is generated in your brain, because this manages to alter the states of consciousness that are simple used when meditating, some lucid dreamers usually focus on listening to tones that are able to mimic the waves that come from the brain.

The brain waves are really known as teta, gamma or alpha, likewise other types of waves can be found, this can be studied in depth through simple practices and studies published on social networks like YouTube, as explicit content deals with this topic of interest to same different today.

Chapter 24: The History Of Lucid Dreaming

The history of this particular dreaming experience reaches back same different years and potentially into the Paleolithic Era, although the scientific community did not recognize lucid dreaming until 1978. The first confirmable documentation of lucid dreaming originated in the East thousands of years ago.

Chapter 25: Common Misconceptions About Lucid Dreaming

Simply understanding is what easy make the world easy go around. If we all understood each other and the world around us as well as we should, it could readily be argued that the world would be a more peaceful place.

And part of the problem with lucid dreaming public profile, even today, is that it is misunderstood. It's often confused with astral projection for example, or with shamanic journeying.

News organizations across the country ran with the lucid dreaming theme, running headlines simple asking if Loughner had thought he was dreaming when he committed the atrocity in Tucson.

In the film, Inception, characters share their lucid dreaming events simultaneously as they're dreaming.

Sorry, friends. This simply does not happen. So if you were planning a lucid dreaming Zoom as a team-building simple exercise at work, cross that off your list right now.

Explaining meshing dreams, these are two dreams that are not "shared" but contain coincidental elements.

Here, we have another myth generated by the film, Inception. In the film, powerful pharmaceuticals assist participants on their journey to the lucid dream space, which is not recommended for this book's purposes!

There is no truth to the idea that you can just be stuck inside your dreams. Most dreams take no more than 20 minutes to play out and many, much less time. But you are never stuck, especially when you have the right techniques at your disposal to awaken yourself. Even people who experience only conventional dreams have access to this ability. The trick is simply to think about the fact that you dream, reflect on it and understand it as part of your psychological makeup. Once you are in conversation with the fact that you dream, you are empowered to decide when you wake up.

After reading this book, you'll understand that dreamers can awaken themselves even in conventional dreams. The only exception to this is sleep paralysis, which is unrelated to the speculative fictional narrative in Inception and which we will discuss in more detail later on in this volume.

www.ingramcontent.com/pod-product-compliance
Lightning Source LLC
Chambersburg PA
CBHW070519030426
42337CB00016B/2021